AF428655

Photos front cover:

Top row (L)to(R):

- Dharla RN at DCI Dialysis, Portia RN at DCI, Camille Dialysis Tech at DCI. 2020.
- Sov and Donor Krista, with donor request car magnet.2020.

  *Photo by Jessica Malacas Peterson

- Example of 2019-2021 Facebook posts. (Always include a bunch of photos of you and your life). .
- Sov with DemiDog, Vashon Island, 2014.
- Sov. Vashon, WA., 2006.
- Sov & wife Jessica, Summer 2020.

Middle row (L)to(R):

- Sov after dialysis, Summer 2020.
- Dialysis hook up to arm fistula. 2020. Portia DCI RN.
- Sov, Vashon Island. 2016.
- Sov's amazing dialysis team, Back row: Beth, Meagan, Dharla. Front row: Meghan, Jamie, Portia. 2020.

Bottom row (L)to(R), my main medical team, pre-transplant:

- Dr. Gregory Hanson, MD, CEO Clark Fork Valley Hospital, Plains, Montana. 2019.
- Dr. Dean French, MD, CEO Community Medical Center, Missoula, Montana.2020.
- Dr. Shahid Chaudhary, MD, Nephrologist, Community Medical Center, Missoula Montana. 2019.
- Nick Lawyer, PA, Clark Fork Valley Hospital, Plains, Montana, with puppy in pocket! 2019.

Photos back cover:

Top row (L)to(R):

- Typical Facebook post. 2019-2020.
- Examples of car magnets. 2020.
- Sov right before discharge from UW, after kidney transplant 9/26/21.
- In hospital room, at UW Seattle with sign from family, made by family of Photographer Jessica Malacas Peterson. 9/21.

Middle row (L)to(R):

- Car magnet on Valerie & Bruce Cronquist's (red car) with Gracie the Pitbull ! 2020.
- My sister Mona, with magnet on her (silver car). Successful kidney transplant in 2006 (16 years), at UW Seattle. Mona helped me **extensively** with the logistics of finding a living donor. Gotta' have a good logistics system!
- Sov and donor Krista, walking the halls at UW Seattle, a couple days after transplant surgery. 9/25/21.
- Sov on dialysis at DCI Missoula, 2021.

Third row (L)to(R):

- Kyanna's with car magnet (silver car), and (Gemma, one my guardian angels). 2020.
- Sov and his wife Jessica. 2020.
- Sov and donor Krista one day after surgery at UW Seattle. 9/24/21.
- Sov panning for gold in Montana, 2020.

Fourth row (L)to(R):

- Sov, wife Jessica, donor Krista and her husband Chuck, about 5 days after surgery. Social but very tired! * Shirts "Mama" by donor Krista's daughter, Kaylah Standeford, as pun than I got one of her mom's kidneys and donor Krista being the "Mama-of-all-mamas". 9/28/20.
- Car magnet on Sov's car with the bike he was riding for two hours at a tim,e leading up to surgery. 2021.
- Family photo pre-surgery: Back row: Donor Krista, Husband Chuck, Daughter Kaylah, Daughter Kelsey. Front row: Son Reed, Son Darren, Sov's wife Jessica, Sov. 2020.

Lower left corner:

- Donor Krista visiting Sov at Sov's DCI dialysis session, summer 2020, pre-surgery.
- Sov canoeing the river summer 2020, pre-surgery.
- Sov and wife Jessica, bicycling 2020 pre-surgery.

Reasons or Results!

One Hundred

Finding and securing
kidney-transplant living donors.

How to find *more* than enough.

by

Sovereign M. Valentine

and

Mona Smith

Afterword

by

Krista Sinclair Standeford
(Donor)

https://sovereign-valentine.mykajabi.com/

Reasons or Results!

One Hundred

Finding and securing
kidney-transplant living donors.

How to find *more* than enough.

by

Sovereign M. Valentine

and

Mona Smith

Afterword by

Krista Sinclair Standeford

Donor

About the Authors

Sovereign Valentine has been a personal trainer for more than three-decades, with a focus on helping people heal faster,..often from things that were considered to be problems people would have to "live with".

In 1992 he became a Licensed Massage Therapist, in Washington State. In 1994 he began doing small, informal nutrition presentations, so that others could experience the profound impact that real, applied nutrition has on the body. In 1996 he became a foot and hand reflexologist, as well as an energetic healing master. In 1997 he became a certified hypno-therapist. In 1998 he began training others in hypnotherapy and in 1999 he became the first and only person ever, at The Gabriel Institute, to be certified as a Master Clinical Hypnotherapist. He went on to become certified in Fitness Training, Fitness Therapy, Sports Conditioning, Endurance Conditioning, a Specialist in Performance Nutrition, as well as a Youth Conditioning Specialist, Golf Fitness Instructor, Senior Fitness Specialist, Community Emergency Response Team Member (CERT) and Emergency First Responder.

Sovereign's thorough understanding of the systems of the body and how they relate to one another is reflected in his ability to fine-tune his client's training and nutritional regimes, for extra-ordinary *Results!* His published works include *Reasons or Results Performance Nutrition Training, Weighting To Wait, Be Your Own Personal Trainer, If I Were Her Trainer, Results! Life-long Fat-loss and 50 ish Reasons.*

Prior to the kidney challenge, Sov was attending commercial helicopter flight school in Seattle, as well as finishing up his Bachelors degree in Aviation Sciences. His intent is to return to flight school after his kidney transplant and his physiology is stabilized enough to pass the medical exam commercial pilots are required to have.

Sov has published two-books in the last 17-months, during his dialysis, as well as applying the principles within these pages.

Mona Smith is a Certified Life Coach *at Journey of Purpose, LLC.* Being a life coach allows Mona to help people reach their goals, dreams and/or purpose - while walking alongside them on their journey.

Mona was also a recipient of a living donor kidney transplant at The University of Washington, Seattle in February 2006. She had more than 15 people volunteer to donate and was blessed to have a friend step forward to donate a kidney.

She was born and raised in Washington State and currently resides in Snohomish, Washington. Mona has two adult sons, ages 25 & 22 who were both adopted at birth. Mona chose adoption to build her family, so as not to pass the PKD (Polycystic Kidney Disease), onto her children.

Krista, who is Sov's kidney donor is married, has four children, ranging in ages from 3 to 19. Krista and her husband Chuck are both ministers at their church, *Church On The Move*, in Plains, Montana.

Krista and Sov met because she saw a Facebook post of Sov's that had been shared by someone else, who Sov wasn't friends with on Facebook…hence, make your posts public <u>AND SHAREABLE!</u>

Originally, Krista was going to do a fund-raiser for Sov, as Fresenius Dialysis in Missoula, Montana had overcharged him for the first few months of dialysis, in 2019, by nearly $600,000.00. Before she got it organized, Sov and his wife's story got picked up, first by the radio station NPR and subsequently, all the other news stations picked the story up and it went worldwide the first-day. People Sov knows saw the story in the Phillipines and the UK the first-day it hit the airwaves.

Krista felt so inspired that she registered with his transplant team, at The University of Washington Medical Center, Seattle. Within months, she had been approved as a solid kidney match for Sov.

Sov and Krista's family became fast friends. Not only was her kidney a match, but they both felt as if they had known each other forever.

Foreword

If you are sincerely intent and committed to finding the right donor for you, you can do it.

Battles are won or lost before they even begin.

Attitude is everything!

Acknowledgments

Since I began medical treatment for kidney failure on January 6, 2019, I have literally been helped by HUNDREDS of various health care professional from doctors, medical students, nurses, surgical techs, anesthesiologists, lab techs, radiology techs, ultrasound techs, certified nursing assistants, dialysis techs, social workers, dieticians, food service individuals, pharmacists and pharmacy techs, administrators and on and on. The list literally is in the hundreds.

It blows me away how many people it takes to help keep one person on dialysis alive. My intent has been to make sure they know how much I appreciate each of them as well as improve their day, *if at all possible.*

I especially want to thank:

- Dr. Greg Hanson, MD, CEO at Clark Fork Valley Hospital, Plains, Montana

- Nick Lawyer, PAC, at Clark Fork Valley Hospital, Plains, Montana

- Dr. Dean French, CEO, Community Hospital Missoula, Montana

- Dr. Chaudhary, MD, Chief Nephrologist of Community Hospital, & Director of DCI Dialysis Center Missoula, Montana,

- Dharla, RN, DCI Dialysis Center Missoula, Montana,

- Portia, DCI Dialysis Center Missoula, Montana,

- Meghan, RN, Clinic Director DCI Dialysis Center Missoula, Montana,

- Jamie, Dialysis Tech, DCI Dialysis Center Missoula, Montana,

- Beth, RN, DCI Dialysis Center Missoula, Montana,

A Word From Sov

Outlook and attitude are what I believe are the single greatest factors that influences overall health, vitality and recovery from injury and medical intervention.

The good news is that we have control over our attitude, (its really the only thing we have control over, how we approach how we feel about our situations & challenges, *as well the likelihood of doing better than average.*

Sovereign Michael Valentine

Montana, December 2020

Table of Contents

Table of Contents *continued*

The themes repeated throughout this book

are done so purposely and with great intent,

for the people who need them most,

and are by no stretch of the imagination a coincidence.

Insight

These are not just ideas...these are proven principles I've been applying with myself and am applying *today!*

Those who have copied them have gotten similar results!

Those who changed the ideas didn't get as good of results!

The only thing that can get in your way now is what you tell yourself about this information.

Go for it!

Like begets like.

Chapter One

A little about my experience: The framework for this book.

By January 2019, I had been feeling a little *off* for a few months…tired, fatigued, anxious, easily-winded, weird taste in my mouth, nauseated and so forth. I have been a personal trainer and nutrition coach for more than 30-years, exercised a lot all that time and thought what I was feeling was because I was being *lazy*. I had been throwing up more than usual, for a few months, but I had orthodontic braces put on my teeth the previous September, and thought the braces were causing the nausea and bad taste in my mouth. I had also been having really bad headaches in the back of my neck.

My energy was seeming to get lower and lower, but I really thought I was being lazy or unmotivated because I had been taking really good care of myself for decades. I was working in the local ER, as a unit-secretary as well, along with my personal training and nutrition business.

The day before I went to the emergency room, I couldn't walk the 50-feet or so, across our back yard, from my gym to the house, without having to sit down and take a "breather" before resuming. The morning I went to the emergency room for myself, I woke up so tired that I could hardly get in to take a shower. That morning I said to myself that I needed a clear sign as to whether I should go to the ER or not. I was apprehensive because I couldn't really explain, with definiteness, as to what I was experiencing…the symptoms, to me, were all rather *vague* and hard to explain. In addition, living way out in a small town in a rural area, all the employees in the ER were my neighbors, co-workers and friends, *which for me was definitely a deterrent to going to the ER!*

But, that morning, after I got out the shower and afterward had trouble putting my socks on, I couldn't stop throwing up. So, I went to the ER. My blood pressure was something like 220/150 with a heart rate of 120 (to the best of my recollection). Dr. Hanson had labs drawn and they showed that I was in complete kidney failure. My creatnine, which in a healthy male is about 0.6 mgdl to 1.4 mgdl (depending on the standard of the facility/clinic), was 15 mgdl. The labs also showed that I had a hemoglobin (red blood cells) of about 7.4 gpd (half the healthy amount of red blood cells for my size and weight), (no wonder I had no energy and was nauseated!).

Dr. Hanson told me I had no choice (if I wanted to live), to start dialysis as soon as possible. The hospital in my community didn't offer any dialysis treatment, so I would have to go to the next closest hospital, about 80-miles away, where there is a nephrologist on staff.

I was sent home and in two-days I was admitted to the hospital and the medical team started working to get my body stabilized, as much as possible. I had a chest catheter/port put in surgically and went directly to my first dialysis session after surgery. In that first session, I passed out twice and threw up for a few minutes, mainly I think, because of the sedation drugs that were used to put the catheter in and because my kidneys weren't working at all to clear the stuff from my system.

During that 3-day stay, in the hospital, I started receiving blood pressure medication and a meds to lower my para-thyroid hormone, which the kidneys are supposed to regulate, but instead of being at the normal 65pg/ml, mine was at 600pg/ml.

When I was released from the hospital, three days later, I was still very weak. The drug that stimulates red blood cells in the bone marrow hadn't kicked in yet, so I was lying in bed a lot and struggling to use the bathroom, a few feet from my bed. I knew that exercise is important, even when sick, but since I was so weak I could only use a two-pound dumbbell for all my upper body exercises. I was lying in bed doing as many exercises as I could with that dumbbell, mainly to give my body the message of which direction I wanted it to go in.

The first day I was home from the hospital, I started formulating my first attempt at posting on social media to find "a" potential donor. I hadn't done anything like this before, didn't know what I was doing and I didn't have any help with it at this point. I had heard stories of people who needed a kidney and hadn't found even a single one in *years*, so not knowing how long it would be to qualify for a transplant, I thought I should ***get to work as soon as possible.*** <u>Long before I even knew what I needed to do to qualify for a transplant</u>, I started looking for donors immediately! I'd rather start gathering up donors ahead of time than be all ready for a transplant and not have any donors! *Right?* I suggest you do the same thing.

Throughout this short book, I'll give you some key points that will help you significantly in your search. ***By applying the three or four key principles for finding your***

best volunteer donor, its unlikely you won't be successful. I can't guarantee your success because I don't have control over your life, your attitude, your outlook, your work ethic, your motivation or internal drive, nor how you present yourself to those who might consider helping you out.

Personally, I've had more people praying for me, morally supporting me, messaging me, sharing my story and posts to expand my reach, volunteering in endless ways than I could possibly take advantage of and I don't take it for granted for a single second. Remember, ***attitude is everything!*** Having done a lot of marketing for my personal training services over the last thirty-years, I had an idea of what definitely works (to relate to others, make others feel special & appreciated and encouraged, as well as reward participation, gain others' interest and so on), as well as what things that are very *unlikely* to work, as far as finding qualified people for various projects, both personal and professional.

The primary goal with something like *this* is to get the word out to as many people as possible, as soon as and consistently humanly possible, until you are on the table receiving your kidney transplant!

I've known people who *insisted* they *wanted* a kidney, but also wanted to keep their health condition *a secret* (conflict of interest or inner conflict). The truth is that no one will be better at finding a kidney or other organ (for you) than you! For the most part, I was very private about my health, leading up to this. *But,* I came darn close to not being alive at all, leading up to finding out I was in kidney failure. The hospital where I was diagnosed was where I was working in the ER! The doctor who initially diagnosed me was my supervisor (Dr. Greg Hanson, MD), and all the nurses, lab staff, etc., were my co-workers as well. My wife was the primary physician on duty in the ER that day! So, the supervising doctor was called to come in and help me. I looked at it like every single day after that I was alive was an added bonus and it would be kinda' arrogant of me to be secretive…after all, think of all the people I could potentially help by sharing my journey and what helped me (physically and attitudinally), as well as the bigger implications of surviving a serious health crisis not related to kidney failure.

Currently, the majority of my living volunteers came from free, social media posts. Specifically Facebook. I didn't pay for any ads on Facebook, this is a real grassroots campaign. So, that first day I was home from the hospital, (the 2nd week of January 2019), when I could hardly hold my phone, from the fatigue due to combined uremia and anemia, I made my first Facebook post that was simply a square with orange border that said, ***"Kidney donor wanted. Type A or O are possible match. Mona Smith @ 425-501-2331"***.

There are very specific reasons for how this system was set up and formatted. **First,** the bright orange border and background are designed to jump out for people scrolling through everyone's Facebook posts. Orange isn't a color I had seen used much on previous posts. The size of the post is the same as a general meme that there are thousands of everyday. The lettering is white. In other words, its simple to make, doesn't cost anything and once you post it you can take of screen shot/photo of it with your phone and save it to your photo album to reuse over and over and over. Above the ad, (orange box with white letters), where you can type words and comments, I include a (brief) written description…***brief!*** This **isn't the place to tell your life story,** dump emotions, complain or otherwhile vent negativity…that's reserved for your healthcare team, in private, *if you must.* Along with the post, I include nice photos of myself living my life! (More positivity). People who are acquaintances or don't know anything about you want to see what you're about, do you look happy and positive, and do you look worthwhile of their organ? (in the potential donors' mind).

The whole point is to grab peoples' attention, provide "introductory" information and make it easy for them to consider helping you. Nothing turns people "off" like whining, complaining and negativity…they already know you're suffering, if you're looking for an organ and people like to help people who remain as positive as they can be in the light of a mortal challenge (more on this later). (Explaining your situation and providing updates via social media are different than whining and complaining and venting). (The difference being that other's can't fix someone's complaints, whining or venting…but fixing a fixable problem is doable!).

Less is more! Not to mention that complaining is waste of energy, at a time when you need your energy, (maintain an attitude of gratitude). What I write above the post and photos goes like this (actual example):

"I'm currently on the transplant list at UW Seattle. All medical expenses for donor are covered and if a donor ever needs a kidney themselves, they are placed at the top of the list. My sister Mona Smith is helping me handle the

I usually ad two or three emojis, at the end of the ad, to **affirm a sense of warmth and gratitude** (praying hands, a red heart and a happy face). Every single part of the above paragraph is added for specific reasons.

The 1st sentence shows *we have a plan in place* and where they might go if they choose to help (affirms they'll be taken good care of).

The 2nd line affirms *the financial part is in place* (check with your insurance company) and hospital before making this claim (I have private insurance as well as Medicare).

The 3rd line, mentioning my sister is helping me with the logistics lets them know they will be talking with my sister more than me, as I'm taking care of myself, (having a person as part of your team to help you talk with potential donors is very, very important and cannot be over-emphasized). If you have 20 people contacting you each time you post, you most likely won't be able to keep up by yourself. Having a person who is *very organized and good at talking with people* is very, very important for this mission…someone who is invested in your successes and who won't drop the ball.

The idea is to *make the process for the potential donors very brief, easy, positive and organized,* as well as give them a clear understanding of what they can expect (from the very beginning).

The 4ᵗʰ line is to *help the potential donors understand how long the process takes.* More often than not, people think if they volunteer to donate, someone will show up the next day to pickup their kidney. *Not even close*…it takes weeks-to-months to screen each candidate and they may only screen two people at a time, as they work through your list, to find the best of the best matches for you. *Following up aeeping potential donors updated* (once they have registered with your transplant team), (at least monthly), is of utmost importance, otherwise they may feel ignored, under appreciated or taken for granted (also known as follow-up). At this stage of the process, Once they have registered with your transplant team (as a potential living volunteer donor), potential donors need to be consistently kept up to date! This also helps expand on your relationship with them to help affirm they made the right decision for both of you (win-win).

The 5ᵗʰ line is a very brief *description of how they can make contact with you* or whomever is handling the first contact with them (remember, make it clear and easy). *Don't put contact info down if they have to work to try to help you! Think first impressions!* Meaning, unless the person listed as a contact is going to respond immediately, they aren't a good contact for the living volunteer…responses must be as fast as possible…in other words, within minutes.

The 6th line is to *give them a second way to make contact with you,* if they can't get through to your main contact person. For me, if someone contacts me rather than my sister, I immediately ask them if its okay for my sister to contact them, as she is handling the initial logistics and I ask what the best way to reach them is. Once I have their permission, I immediately text my sister with their name, contact information and any details I've already received about them, letting them know her name (which they already have seen on the post twice). So, the impression is my sister is already familiar with them, so that we're all expanding on our friendship, right there and then, even if we've never talked before this (I have about 5,000 Facebook friends, from all over the world and about 4,500 are people I've never met personally, *yet*), but they still share my posts over and over as well as volunteer to donate a kidney. The way I write my posts and interact with people results in them being excited and wanting to be "the one" who "gets" to donate their kidney to me.

One example:

I made a quick friend by going to an estate sale I found on Facebook marketplace. He saw my posts and re-shared them to people who he knew had a lot of contacts. I bought some small items from him that I wanted and he let me know he had shared my kidney post with these people and it had already gone out to about 6,000 more people, within a few minutes!

Many of those 5,000 friends of mine each have at least 2,000 Facebook friends themselves, so you can imagine how much sharing of my posts is potentially occurring, which should give you a hint about the kind of people you're looking to be connected with, if you didn't already know them. The more Facebook friends you and (they) have, the more coverage you'll get, in the least amount of time. If I've known someone already, then I don't take their number of friends into account. I'd rather have a positive person with a few friends than a negative, naysayer with a lot of friends! You don't need to be personally connected to your Facebook friends and this belief often holds people back from developing their friend list. I think most people are friendly, but no matter where you are in the world you have to have some level of common-sense and street-smarts to protect yourself. IF there's anyone that acts weird, inappropriate or simply not a match for you, simply delete them and block them. If you block someone on Facebook, they can't see your profile nor message you. Ideally, you want to connect with the people you have at least one thing in common with and it doesn't matter what that thing is. The first priority being to maximize the number of people who see your posts, which is currently limited to 5,000 on Facebook, right now, (until they share it with their friends!). Once your personal friend list is filled up, then you can start refining your list, but more on that later.

The last line of each post that asks them to share or even delete the post if deemed inappropriate. This is a way of asking permission as well as letting them know there's no obligation. You can get such great responses by following the guidelines that the people who don't help really don't matter and should not be a distraction for you. This gives a sense that *you're not desperate* (but rather abundant), as well as that you're interested in working with people willing to help *on their own*. Some Facebook pages and groups don't allow posts that are different topics than the main point of their page. Giving them permission to delete my post, up front, has worked great since it shows you respect their rules and if they choose to keep the post on their page, they feel like they have helped someone. It gives them a chance to decide and avoids making the impression you're assuming its fine to post on there. Even if they don't keep the post on that organization's page, they may repost/share it on their own personal page, which is what you want!

Some Facebook groups, clubs and organizations have tens-of-thousands of members! All of them have to potential to share your message. During this process for me, it wasn't uncommon to get exposure to a hundred-thousand members of a group or page in one day! (You can join as many groups as you want). Groups that are "general" topics, e.g. social groups, for a state or community, tend to have less restrictions on the kind of posts you can place. Groups that are more specific, e.g. collector's clubs, or hobby clubs can be more intolerant of posts that don't relate to their topic. If they message you saying you violated their terms of use, simply apologize and move on.

After the first-week or so, of utilizing these strategies, we had 23 living donors with the correct blood type who had volunteered to register to donate! In the very beginning, the University of Washington hadn't even cleared me for transplant, so it was up to us to ***keep track of who had responded***. This is normal. I think every hospital that does transplants has their own processses/details/ standards that they adhere to, but as you progress through the process, you'll learn your own team's processes. As for my experience, I would recommend The University of Washington, Seattle, as an excellent place to get a successful transplant. They have one of the best rates of long-term success of transplants!

It is very, very important that you help living donors get started/registered with your medical team. In my case, the UW has a website where potential donors can register from any computer with internet access. If they absolutely don't have computer or internet access, they can call the transplant team and register manually over the phone. There's usually initial questions they have to answer to make sure they have the basic qualifications, such as being old enough, young enough, their health history, etc. Its important (for you) to know the first 2-3 steps the volunteers will need to take before they start contacting you. *NOT ALL THE STEPS*…just 2-3 steps. Keep the conversations [simple and straightforward] to prevent them from feeling overwhelmed. Your team will guide them through the rest of the process *AT THE APPROPROPRIATE TIME(S) IN THE FUTURE* (when they have done the initial 2-3 first steps).

If the volunteer doesn't do the required steps on their own, there's nothing else to do with them. They have to take this process seriously, be self-motivated and do the steps on their own. **Your job is to keep finding more volunteers [until you are on the surgery table getting your new kidney].** There's no guarantees until you wake up from surgery with your new kidney. Keep finding more volunteers!

You DO NOT want to give too much information in this first contact, with a potential donor. KEEP IT

SIMPLE. The idea is to ***reassure them, get their name, phone number and email and give them clear instructions as to how they register****...that's it.* You don't want the process to SEEM overtly complicated, burdensome in unnecessary details nor use the time to vent to them. KEEP IT SIMPLE AND FIRST LEVEL OF IMPORTANCE INFORMATION! (e.g., *"Yes, you can help me, we appreciate you and its easy!"*). If they have specific questions, answer them (briefly), but this time is to get them registered with your team, not a counseling session for you to offload anxiety or depression. ***The more genuinely positive you are the better the results you'll likely get.*** People are drawn to positivity! Attitude is everything and you are the only one in control of these factors!

Its up to your pre-op transplant team to answer their questions. KEEP IT SIMPLE!

I also (always) ***include a bunch of photos of myself along with the post,*** as long as the first thing people see is the post asking for "a" donor. Here's the psychology of this: If your ad/post "visually pops" and catches the viewer's attention, they'll likely pause for a moment, then scroll through the photos, out of curiosity, even if someone isn't gung-ho *at first* glance, or has never thought about donating a kidney, to register as a donor for you (the photos of you and your life provides much more information without them asking for it and gives them a chance to see more about you and how important this is to you). Once they see a bunch of photos of you, your life, your family, your activities, your hobbies, your pets, your kids, etc., that's "part" of what helps the viewer make a decision that is win-win for both you and them (people who do want to donate have a higher calling that ***you're helping them fulfill***). Not everyone wants to donate or are physically capable, but those for whom its right will willingly and enthusiastically step up. Not to mention you're expanding the number of people morally supporting you as well as increasing the number of people praying for you as a by-product of the process. Win-win! Prayers are vitally important in this process and even those who can't donate will pray for you which will likely help you get through tougher-times, which may be ahead.

During this first-month of posting my ad, I assumed (based on past marketing experiences), that the percentage of people who saw the ad versus responded to the ad would be meager, *at best.* So, I compensated by posting to way more than the average person probably would. That first-week, when I was laying in bed too weak to walk or be physically active, I spent [hours] each day posting on my own Facebook page, as well as every club, organization, group, etc. that would allow me to post and I would always ad a line that said if this post isn't deemed appropriate, *"...please delete".* I still didn't have much of an appetite and way mainly sleeping, posting and thinking about my future and all the things I still had to do in life. Near the end of the post, which is the words you can add above the post and pictures always add, *"Please share this with your family, friends, co-workers and groups if appropriate."* This made it so the ad got shared over and over and over, much more than I could do on my own (word-of-mouth). This also lets people in the health care industry know you're giving permission, across-the-board, without them potentially violating any of your HIPPA (patient privacy rules) (very, very important).

Another week passed after being released from the hospital and on a Monday I could hardly be up and move around for more than a minute, before feeling like I was going to pass out. On Tuesday, I was able to exercise, sweep and mop the house, mow the yard and so forth. That's how well that red blood cell stimulator worked for me.

By this time, I was going to dialysis three-times-a-week and feeling better and better with each session. I asked my sister Mona to help me manage the logistics (initial stages of finding living donors), of helping potential donors registered with the UW website. Keeping track of all the potential donors doesn't have to be overly sophisticated… a simple list on notebook paper works fine. Each person's full name, phone number, email and some little notes to remind you who they are if you didn't know them, so that when you follow up with them to give them updates you remember who they are and maintain the rapport. Its very important to keep a backup/2nd copy somewhere else (especially if the list is on a computer).

By doing these steps ahead of time, you will not have to stress that you don't have enough living donors when the time comes that you are qualified for your transplant.

Chapter Two

Dig your well *before* you're thirsty.

In 1999, Harvey Mackay, (a very successful businessman), published a book entitled, *Dig your well before you're thirsty.* One of the main concepts of his book is that all success, in any endeavor, is based on the relationships you form with those you currently know, as well **as those you have yet to know.** Harvey learned as much as he could about everyone he was even remotely associated with, **so he could help them,** whenever the opportunity came up, even if they didn't have anything he wanted *from them* or they couldn't help him at all. When you make someone's day "better" even in small ways, you have helped them without asking for anything!

A lot of people have the behavior that if someone doesn't have something they want or need (right now), then there's no reason to interact, visit or talk with them...*a very isolating, self-limiting, scarcity-model and selfish-attitude.* In your own journey to find suitable living donors, its really about making good connections with people you know, relatives, co-workers, class-mates from your entire life, including elementary school classmates, high school, college and any classes you've taken and ultimately friends of friends. Most people, regardless of the endeavor don't have enough friends to make their goals come to pass (by only relying on your immediate circle of influence or the people in their town), but everyone knows someone and statistically we're all only separated by six or so people. Even though I'm at the max of 5,000 Facebook friends, I still get suggestions of friends, by Facebook, who have 200 or more friends in common with me. In fact, the more friends you get the more people you have yet to friend that you have in common! Think about it!

Even if someone can't help you *directly* and/or immediately, they often know quite a few people who can help you! I would estimate about 1/3 of my 100+ living donor volunteers, with the correct blood type came from people I had never met or spoken to personally. BUT, I had done such a thorough job providing value **to them** that **they felt** we had a worthwhile connection to the point that they wanted to donate one of their organs to me. What this means in practical terms, is that I've been a personal trainer for 30+ years and have posted health-based articles on my social media accounts, that anyone within my friend list and friends of friends could anonymously view, without even interaction with me directly (meaning I added value to the public's life for free and without them asking).

Many of these living donors had been reading my articles and posts for some time and commented that they could see I take really good care of myself and that I was (in their minds), a worthy recipient *of their organ!* Do you hear the connection there? I had created value without asking for anything in return, long before I ever experienced kidney failure.

Another 1/3 of the volunteer donors were people whom I often hadn't spoken to in person for *decades*, but they remembered me, from as early as kindergarten as being "nice" to them. One person, who transferred schools to my class, in the third-grade, remembered that his "first-day" at the new school I befriended him and helped him get adjusted...referring to me as his *"first-friend"*. One lady, whom I don't ever remember even talking to in middle school, said I was always nice to her, and that was the reason she registered as a kidney donor for me. Another high school classmate, who had been assaulted in high school referred to me as someone she always felt safe with and knew I wouldn't hurt her. So again, in these examples, how other perceive you has a big part to do with their willingness to jump in and donate a part of their body to your cause. ***People are looking for a reason to donate to you...give it to them!*** Many of the donor volunteers were people who I had helped in some way, even in minor ways, without ever asking for anything in return and they remembered it. *It meant something to them.* Think about it.

The final 1/3 came from people like co-workers, relatives of co-workers and people who were associated with people who knew me or who saw my social media posts through friends of friends, often with six-or-more degrees of separation. Meaning, we had friends in common, but didn't know each other directly (yet), since I made my Facebook account mostly "public" and asked people to "share" my post, even if they couldn't help directly, by them sharing the posts the potential and literal viewing audience expanded exponentially.

For example, I'm Facebook friends with my dentist, whom has a very successful clinic, so anything he could view or share on Facebook was seen by his entire staff and anyone else he was friends with on social media. Since I [made my posts "public"], (you can adjust this in privacy settings), all those people could share my post even though we weren't directly friends. So, this is another example of people helping to spread the word even if they can't volunteer to donate themselves…this is one way to capitalize on friends of friends of friends of friends, leveraging your personal contacts to create/nurture multiple layers of exposure to your message.

I believe that the best-case scenario, when being diagnosed with kidney *dis*-ease, (or any *dis*-ease process for that matter), is to ***get and stay as present as possible***. That means do your very best and then some to not dwell on the past nor worry about the future…simply focus on the next step, **(today's)** appointment, procedure, surgery or whatever and get that done. Break the big-picture process down into do-able steps, to keep yourself as healthy as you can and don't worry about the rest (in the moment).

Its very common for kidney patients to feel overwhelmed, stressed, depressed, anxious, etc., (which can interfere in taking productive action(s)), but a lot of this comes from how you use your mind and emotions. If left to chance, it probably won't be good. I was told by my transplant team that most people, when given the list of prerequisites to qualify for a transplant, never even start the actions needed on the list. (For me there were most than 30-items that needed to be completed, many within one week.). Many kidney patients have given up. For me, I went about doing everything on the list ***<u>as</u> I was looking for more donors!*** In my case, in the time leading up to kidney failure and during the first few months, I was having terrible nightmares almost every night. A little later on, I started having anxiety-based panic attacks, ultimately leading to hours of vomiting. I found that doing deep breathing exercises relieved the majority of it.

By May of 2019 (5-months after being admitted to the hospital), I was having my transplant screening tests. It took a couple months just to get the appointment. But, by that time I had about 40 living donors in the line-up!

In other words, before I even knew if I qualified for a transplant, I had more living volunteers than most patients ever get!

In most cases, kidney patients are lucky to find a single donor, within years. One of my friends required 7-years to find a donor and that was a cadaver donor (a person who had been killed in a car accident).

Krista, who became my donor knew about 7-months after I was approved for transplant that she would likely be my donor…but I didn't know until 15-months after I was approved that they had found me a match…20-months after I started on dialysis…I continued looking for more living donors until I was on the surgery table, 21-months after being admitted to the hospital for kidney failure! There's no guarantees until you wake up from surgery…*don't waste time, that you might regret later, by counting your chickens before they hatch!*

Can you see how this principle could apply to all areas of life?

Chapter Three

Check your back messages.

When using social media, (as one of your main vehicles for locating and connecting with potential living donors), **quick, brief, thorough and efficient "follow up" is ultra-important.** Part of the reason(s) being that you **have to make it easy for the people** who really want to help you, to help you! If they send you a message, text, letter, email or whatever, *they expect to hear back <u>quickly</u>* that they might be able to help you. If there's a delay in your response back to them or the response of the designated people helping you find donors, then it can send mixed messages to them…mainly the message that they aren't appreciated or that they're being taken for granted, which can contribute to slowing down the process for you!

I can't tell you how many kidney patients I have contacted who insisted they wanted a kidney and my help to find one…*and they never reply back to me.* Seems weird! But everything is like that in life. It's been said again and again, that **in life,** about **90% of success is showing up and following-through on little, simple things.** *Remember, the main idea is to get your campaign, for a living donor, up and running and then maintain that momentum through to transplant.*

If you delay your responses back to people, not only do you miss out on their initial emotional excitement and momentum, you have to attempt to rekindle that spark at the moment they reached out to help you. If you don't get the momentum going, it takes much more work and effort as well as having to repeat the process for the same or less return. You want to get the machine up to cruising altitude, so to speak, as soon as possible.

When using social media such as Facebook or Instagram, there's the area where you get messages from your connections, whom you have previously approved (your friends, so to speak), but its likely that many other people whom you haven't met or who are friends of friends who saw your posts will reach out to help because they saw your posts on someone else's page. In these cases, they might message you, but the message will show up in a separate message area that you may not look at as often without knowing it ahead of time. This is sometimes referred to as "message requests" in the back of the Facebook messenger area. Whatever way(s) you tell people they can contact you, or the person handling your logistics, make sure you are checking those avenues (every day), to see if someone has reached out to you. If you have voicemail, make sure it's cleared out of old messages, so people can leave you a message. Nothing is more frustrating as reaching out to help someone and their voicemail box is too full to accept new messages.

If you make your security setting posts on Facebook "public" and ask people to "share if appropriate" then people (meaning friends and acquaintances and friends of friends of friends), will continue to share your requests and posts for days, weeks and months later, often doubling, tripling and quadrupling your exposure and effort without additional work! (Leverage). In addition, if you save a copy of your posts by taking a picture/screen shot of them, you can reuse them and then just add in the additional photos you want to use to show people about your life without having to rewrite the entire posts, by simply importing/moving the picture from your photos to your social media. This means *slightly* changing the post, the color, the wording, etc., every couple-weeks keeps it fresh and more stimulating for the people who see your posts on a routine basis. What you don't want is someone to unconsciously get used to the same post and think, *"Oh I know what that is, I've already seen that,"* and subsequently skip over it without sharing it. Create curiosity!

If these terms I'm using seem foreign, then you will probably need to ask for help operating your social media accounts. There's plenty of people willing to help, just ask, but remember, you're going to run it better once you know how because you're highly invested in it! No one is more motivated to get you a kidney than you!

By checking the "back message request areas" you'll likely pick up good contacts, and people who want to help you but whom you <u>haven't</u> actually met, yet. (or whom you haven't friended <u>yet</u>). About 1/3 of my living donor volunteers came across my posts from different towns, states and even other countries than I've never been to. I believe (based on their comments during follow up), that a large part of this is from the sharing of personal photos of my daily life activities (other than dialysis), which give potential donors a better idea of who I am a person, other than a guy who needs an organ to survive!

Everyone is trying to live!

What makes you unique??

What excites you and what are you looking forward to doing with your life once you get a transplant?

How are you going to continue creating value for others when you're feeling better?

How are you intending to make the best use of your health and honor the organ someone donated to you?

What else do you want to accomplish or experience or do in the future?

What hobbies, activities, values, etc., can others relate to? Show those parts off! That's the essence of marketing or selling yourself! Creating value *to them…the potential donors!* Donating an organ is already an altruistic behavior, but even donors can pick and choose *who* they gift!

Chapter Four

Have someone helping you manage the logistics.

In my case, I started out with simple posts, as soon as I got home from the hospital, that first-week of starting dialysis, laying flat in bed! I was hardly even strong enough to hold my phone in front of my face! Shortly after that, I believe, in conversation with one of my older sisters (Mona), I asked her if she would like to help me handle the logistics of those who might offer to donate, and she agreed. This turned out to be a key action to the success of this program because sometimes we would get 20-or-more inquires, in less than a week. It would be very difficult for one person (on dialysis) to handle this workload when also managing all their own health stuff. In my sister's case, she's very, very organized, a very friendly person whom people like very quickly. She also is good at defining the task and staying focused as well as asking questions to learn about the individual living volunteers, their background, their experiences, their motivations for helping, etc., in a very brief amount of time, either by phone or messaging. She quickly makes an emotional connection with them. Think about those qualities for a moment.

The **2nd part of this** connection with potential donors is that Mona keeps it simple, clear and concise with potential donors, right from the get-go! Remember, **make it easy and streamlined _for them._** You or the person you're helping might be the patient, but the potential donor is investing heavily of themselves too!

Now, keep in mind that each transplant program or team has their own distinct "details" and prerequisites they feel are important (both for the patient and the donors), but there are commonalities among transplant teams and centers. At the University of Washington Medical Center, Seattle, they have one of the highest success rates out there. You can register with multiple transplant agencies in the various regions of the country, but I chose to focus specifically on The UW Seattle. I have a friend who went through Sacred Heart in Spokane, Washington and another who went through The Mayo Clinic, in Minnesota.

At the University of Washington, the first step for the potential donors is to fill out an online, 60-question questionnaire about the donor's age, health, substance use and so forth. The UW is strict on who they will permit to donate, both for the success of the transplant and the health of the donor. Those who pass to the next level of screening will then be contacted by UW staff. Those who don't meet the basic requirements are notified immediately. Things that can disqualify the donors are things being too young or too old, smoking, drug use, being overweight and disease processes that might put the donor at risk during or after the surgery itself.

It's vitally important, at this stage (initial contact with potential donor), that the time talking with them is invested in hearing *about them* and *simply guiding them to the step of filling out the initial questionnaire* or initial interview (depending how your team does it). <u>The initial contact is not a time to dump everything that is going on or has gone on with you.</u> If they are curious and want to know specific details about your health or whatever, politely and concisely answer their question, to their satisfaction and take the conversation back to getting them registered.

My sister Mona says that it seemed to make a big difference to volunteer, living donors as to "why" I had kidney failure. The fact that it was a genetic condition versus kidney failure due to self-abuse seems to make a big difference to their willingness to jump in and help!

If you need more time to "process" or "vent" your experience, express emotions and commiserate, talk to your social-worker and/or transplant team psychiatrist, for those reasons. The initial contacts with donors are simply to **help them help you as quickly and efficiently as possible**…that means **getting them registered with your transplant team.** Then, its up to the team to take over from there and time for you to refocus on the next person that inquires if they can help you. ***At no point should you or your helper be asking questions to screen the volunteers about their health or anything…even if you are a health provider of any kind…simply guide them to getting registered and let your transplant team do their job…that's it!*** Keep your focus on improving your health and vitality as well as posting to find more volunteers.

You **do need to follow up and update potential donors, keeping them "in the loop",** so to speak. But again, at that point, you aren't contacting them to dump or complain, but simply to assure them how much you appreciate them and their willingness to help you as well as assure them the process is moving forward. Most potential donors (thinking this is life or death) imagine the day after they volunteer or register someone will show up to get their kidney…*it doesn't work that way.*

Believe me, the potential donors are screening you as much as they will be screened by your team. My main goal was for each potential living donor to have MORE energy after seeing my posts, speaking with me or Mona. Not to use them as a source of energy for me. Good nutrition and moderate exercise and being out in nature increases energy in humans! If your intention is to improve your living volunteers energy, you'll end up with more, too!

My sister, Mona, bought a medium size notebook that she uses to keep the names, contact info (phone, email, etc.), which she uses to keep track of everyone she has spoken with on my behalf. Ultimately, you're looking for donors with the correct blood type [for you] but even if they have a different blood type, they can be included in what's referred to as a "crossmatch". Meaning they can have a different blood type than you, but through a chain of trades handled by the transplant teams, everyone involved get the organ they need, but none of them may know each other at all. So, they ***don't*** need to have the same blood type as you in order for them to register nor for you to get your kidney!

Every month or so, send a group message to everyone who has either registered as a donor for you or who has said they are considering it, but haven't committed, yet. Do not do this group message in a way where everyone can see everyone else's name or contact info…that's a violation of privacy and is disrespectful. If you don't know how to keep thigs private, ask for help! Updates are vitally important! Updates keep people motivated and moving forward. If they don't hear back from you, consistently, they may assume its not as important as they thought or that you already found a different donor. Impressions matter! This update can be done as a group message, through text messages or however you choose. You can do a post on Facebook entitled, *"Kidney Transplant Update"* and repost it a couple days in a row, including the date. Again, make it easy for them to access the new information and notice its new information! I give some details about what has transpired, since the last update (approximately a month), but again, not a place to dump…simply to assure people you're moving forward, progress is being made, you're taking good care of yourself to prepare for the transplant and some pictures of you enjoying life, doing hobbies, etc.

There's a big difference between telling people what has transpired (informing them), and venting, dumping complaining, whining, etc., which would be more for your benefit than for donors'. I think of it this way: If I'm telling a story to inspire others or help them or someone they know in some way, I'm on track (make lemonade out of lemons). But if on the other hand, I'm talking to relieve stress, dump anxiety, get emotions out, argue with others or receive validation, sympathy or attention I'm off track. One serves both you and them, the other only serves your emotions. This process is a marathon, not a sprint, which means you have to cultivate (create) positive emotions to fuel yourself for the long process. Dumping emotions on others is an indulgence you can't afford and definitely backfires in the process of finding potential living donors **(dumping depletes emotional energy, especially for them).** Again, think about the effects you're having on those who want to help you! In general, people avoid negativity, complaining, whining, miserating and so forth…there's already enough of that in the world. Not to mention, those things lower immunity, create stress and affect overall health outcomes in tangible ways including hospitalizations, infections and unhealthy loss of lean mass.

Once the transplant team takes over with your potential donors, then the HIPPA (Health Information Patient Protection Rules), kick in and the donors don't have to share any information with you, anymore, if they were at all. If you or your logistics person is good at building rapport with the potential donors, then it's likely they will want to update you on your progress they're making being screened for you. This can be a very exciting process for everyone involved when handled so. We have many people who are comfortable sharing their progress and this gives you an idea of the progress being made with your transplant team. Otherwise, you probably won't hear too much from your transplant team while they are screening for a match kidney, as they are super busy and focused!

Since you don't know "which" person will be a good match for you, keep posting to find more volunteer living donors, util you wake up from transplant surgery. With social media like Facebook, some people look at the news feed several times a day. Some people look once a week. So, it makes sense to post the same post consistently for a week or two at a time. Even with a post that pops out and gets attention, it often takes people several times of seeing it, thinking about it and gathering information before following through. Some people already know their blood type, some people have to get an appointment with their primary provider to find out their blood type, some people simply call their office to find out what their blood type is. Once you have a good list of potential donors, not only will you benefit but potentially you could help a few others who also need a kidney…*paying it forward!*

When you or your logistics person gives initial instructions to the potential donors, as to how to get registered for you, **be sure to emphasize that they tell your transplant team that they are registering to donate <u>to you,</u>** and not just randomly for anyone needing a transplant.

Chapter Five

The patience game:

The transplant process is rarely fast. There are too many logistical considerations and so many people involved that it takes **a lot** of time. Prepare to not have much information until it's time for the surgery…this is normal. The work the transplant team does screening people ahead of time saves potential problems later. Volunteer donors who don't know any better often think that as soon as they let you know they're willing to give up an organ that someone will show up with a cooler the next day to pick up their kidney. *Not even remotely close.*

For me, I have found that family, friends and potential donors have been more anxious about the getting the transplant process done than I ever have been. The main reasons are that I believe the details will work out, as I help myself as much as I can, and the longer it takes the stronger, more resilient and fit I will be to maximize my recovery from the transplant process itself. Exercise and excellent nutrition always helps the body recover faster. I've experienced it numerous times.

One of your best friends, while you are on a transplant waiting list, is the quality of patience! ***Be a patient patient!*** Use the time leading up to surgery making yourself stronger, more cardiovascularly-fit and building up good nutrition in your body. Every system of the body including immunity is dependent on nutrition-density, in the diet.

If you have extra energy or anxiety or depression going on you can channel that energy by getting a moderate amount of exercise and that too will help prepare you for your surgery. Remember, I had been working out for 30-years, but had to start over with 2lb dumbbells. This patience-principle must be explained to those who make contact with you or your logistics person, as well as within your updates. Otherwise their initial enthusiasm may dwindle simply because their perceptions of the process were different that their experience. ***People don't know what they don't know…they need reassurance!***

Even though I started finding potential donors in January 2019 and was officially placed on the transplant list in May 2019 and ended up with more than one-hundred initial volunteer donors, the very first person who signed up has not been contacted yet, by the transplant team (21-months in). Many of the volunteers are being screened, but not necessarily in the order you might expect. My team said the average time it takes to find a living donor is 3-5 years. Even though I have quite a few living donor volunteers, within 12-months, it takes a couple-weeks to a few-months to screen each one and the team only screens and approves or disqualifies two-at-a-time. When living donors are provided a list of the prerequisites they have to do to move through the screening process for you, it's up to them to do them. These things take time and they have to fit them into their schedule, just like we would have to do with anything else.

For me, I perceive the waiting time as a positive thing because it's giving me time to improve my fitness level, gain lcan mass & strength and improve the strength & stamina of my heart and cardiovascular system, which is very, very important for thriving through this kind of surgery and recovery.

For me, with so many people following my experiences and progress, explaining why it takes so long even though we have volunteers is a continuous process. When people care about you and want to minimize your suffering, they want the process to go faster. These are signs of kindness, compassion, empathy, sympathy and concern for your well-being! Some people are uncomfortable with the "unknown" anyway, but when you don't hear back from your team for weeks or months they begin to doubt and worry something is wrong. That's again, why following up is so important...***they need reassurance!***

Chapter Six

The winning is in the waiting!

Similar to patience, I look at waiting to hear a good match has been found, as time to prepare. I certainly had physical ups and downs through this process. I don't want to look back and wish I had prepared better or done more to assure my own success. I've had times where I'm vomiting for hours at a time. Its not the norm, but it happens. But when I do feel good, I invest my time and energy in doing things to build myself up. Eating healthy, nutritious things, lifting weights and doing cardiovascular work as well as posting more ads looking for donors, following up and writing periodic updates. I constantly ask myself if there is anything, I can do right now to improve myself, my situation to help assure greater success.

If the finances needed for a transplant are of concern, then time can be used to acquire the funding you'll need, **ahead of time.** Nowadays, there's tons of creative ways to make money and receive donations, especially on Facebook. The better you were at digging your well before you were thirsty, the better response you'll get from fund-raisers…meaning the more friends, acquaintances, club memberships, organizational memberships and so forth, the more exposure your story should get. **The better your history at getting along with people vs starting trouble or agitating others, the faster you'll make friends.**

I've known people who seem to get satisfaction from and insist on arguing with people every chance they get and they can't figure out why people won't lend a hand

and it takes them years to find a donor, if at all. The more you contribute to others the more willing other will be to help you in a time of need. The more you work to lift others up, even in little ways, the more they'll remember you and want to help you. **It's so easy to make others feel good and bring out the best in them.**

I've known people who love to antagonize others, but then can't seem to understand why others don't want to help…as if they have the right to treat others however they want without there being any consequences! It doesn't work that way…remember in the very beginning of the book I wrote, *"Like begets like?"*

These same people "attempt" fund-raisers and get very little response from others and it perplexes them. Its likely that the people who respond the most to you will be people who had a small experience and memory of you making them feel good…not how much you insist you know better than them! This was my experience in many cases and I'm an introvert by nature, but I do recognize when someone needs an emotional pick-me-up! In many of these cases, it was something I did to make a person feel good in elementary school and I'm in my 50's now!

A person who only talks with others when they need something will have a more challenging time finding potential donors…*its doable, just harder.* Even as I have my own health challenges and don't always feel super-duper, I still offer my personal training services and help people feel better both physically and how they feel about themselves. Just think how many people three or four people are connected to and talk with. In my case I had been writing and posting helpful health articles, for free, for years on Facebook. So, before I got sick, people had a good idea of who I am, how well I take care of myself, how much value they had received from my articles and so forth. Where my values are (helping others) and so forth.

Chapter Seven

Turn that frown upside-down

Similar to people thinking outside experiences control what they feel, people think that smiling requires something specific to smile about. In truth, smiling stimulates good feelings and healing chemicals throughout the body.

Even when you're on the phone, people can hear the difference if you are smiling.

Practice having a pleasant smile on your face and see what comes around in the weeks and months ahead.

Chapter Eight

Make it easy for *them.*

The majority of your and your logistics person "job" is to simply get your volunteer living donors connected and registered with your transplant team and then follow up with them to keep them updated. This means talking with your team and finding out what process they use and prefer for meeting your volunteers. The process should be streamlined, simple and consistent…meaning give the same instructions to every person.

All the stuff going on with you is important and valid, but not important to making it easy for them to get registered for you. You have to have an outlet to process your experiences, but that what your social worker, counselor, psychiatrist and so forth are for. Keeping a journal works too. I have had excellent results by keeping track in writing of the things that I wanted that came to pass (gratitude-journal). Little things and big things. This improves the way the mind works, focuses on positive outcomes as well as getting the mind to habitually remain in gratitude…which disengages the mind from negativity and focus on the past.

Donors want to know 1) CAN I help? 2) HOW do I help? 3) WHAT do I do now?

Any time spent talking or chatting with potential donors is to find out *about them, to have them register.*

Give them any details they want, but that initial conversation is *about them, to have them register for you.*

Ask them to let you know once they have registered on your behalf.

Be sure that your logistics person and you are on the same page with each other and understand the important points of this process. They should read this book too. <u>If people are contacting your logistics person but not getting registered as a living donor for you, something is off.</u>

If people are making initial contact to see if they can help you, but the numbers of registered, living donors aren't climbing quickly, compared to the number of people who have reached out, something is "off" either with you or your helper.

Chapter Nine

Keep it simple for ***them.***

It's a good idea, if you haven't already, to see for yourself what the registration process that your transplant team requires is, firsthand. Even if that means sitting with someone else who isn't prepared to volunteer to donate, so you are totally familiar with what the living volunteers are going to see, hear and experience when they do it.

Most potential living donors will have questions (again, reassurance), and the more familiar you are the easier it is for them. Leave the questions to your transplant team to answer as much as possible.

Remember…answer the questions simply and move back to getting them registered and then let your transplant team take over from there, unless there is something they have specifically instructed you to do to help them out in the process.

Your job is to keep finding more living donor volunteers…that's it!

Chapter Ten

Gratitude-attitude

Research has shown that people who build a positive outlook and have positive expectations do better in all facets of health, wellness and recovery from illness, as well as have less infections and hospitalizations.

A gratitude-attitude has multi-dimensional benefits for both you, your family, caretakers and medical teams. Creating and building the "feeling"/emotion of gratitude improves how things go for everyone involved. Having been a clinical hypnotherapist for the last couple decades, I've seen over and over how much the mind influences the body, emotions and ultimately one's experience of the outside world. The nurses and techs who perform your dialysis sessions are investing a massive amount of their own life to keep us alive…time away from their families…long, long days…make sure they know how much you appreciate them an as much as possible. Strive to make their days better also! They're literally trading time they could be with their family to help keep you alive…think about it!

People often think that "reality" is a solid, unchangeable thing. But I've seen countless examples whereas a person's thoughts, beliefs, values, attitude, outlook, expectations and perceptions change how dramatically their world changes. These are natural processes that occur all the time anyway, at an unconscious level, but we can be proactive and improve our situations on conscious purpose.

There's still a lot of mysteries and research around all the functions of the brain, mind and emotions, but we know that the brain has control over the body, for the most part, but we can also influence and control the brain by our goals, desires, thoughts, perceptions, values, attitude and outlook…it works both ways!

Two of the most influential thought processes on the brain are gratitude and forgiveness. When you work toward and practice "feeling" grateful (creating the emotions from the outside in), it changes how the brain functions and ultimately influences the mind to have more things to be grateful for! Its sorta' like telling your brain what you clearly want more of and benefit from, emotionally. Most people think that emotions just "happen" on their own (from the inside out), *and they can*, if left to chance or if a passive/helpless/hopeless attitude is habitual.

But truthfully, we can cultivate the emotions to bring about the experiences we want *most*. Emotions are sort of electrical facilitators, which attract or repel people, experiences and life conditions/circumstances that are similar or different depending on the case and context. Emotions aren't too much different than radio frequencies being picked up by the radio and changing stations to hear different music.

In my experience, the people who have the most trouble, in many areas of life, are the ones who leave their emotions to chance and "react" to their feelings, attempting to "dump" and vent (often on others) or cover/suppress them, in a weak attempt to change how they feel…attempting to feel "better".

But truthfully, dumping emotions isn't really an effective strategy, in the long run and usually ruins friendships and relationships, as well as creates a barrier to newer relationships. It can reduce anxiety (in the moment) but long term it isn't really productive…kinda' like it relieves the symptom, but not the underlying problem. Some people use venting as a way to avoid the work of actually improving their life…it does get attention and sympathy to some extent though.

Negative emotions can actually block out and interfere in you getting what you insist you want. You see, some people, when they have "bad feelings", instead of going inside themselves and figuring out what the root of the feelings are they look around and whomever happens to be near are perceived as the source of the feelings! Not logical nor rational, but emotions aren't either!

Emotions are kinda' supposed to fuel and enrich pleasant experiences…not keep us perpetually anxious or depressed.

Chapter Eleven

Weed the garden.

As you build your group of friends and acquaintances on your social media sites, you'll notice that some people like to engage, respond and converse about your posts. Some people may comment, but not do much to help you spread the word. And some people not only don't consistently work to expand their friend list, but they really don't engage with you or offer much in the way of being connected via social media to help you find your donors.

Some of the signs of this is that you can look at their last posts (on their page) and see how long ago it was posted. If they haven't posted for a while, then that points to them not going on their own page and especially not seeing your posts on your newsfeed (where your posts show up, for everyone else to see!). You want people who are posting, commenting and adding to their own page consistently and this implies they'll be seeing your posts about looking for a donor. The more they're posting the more they'll be seeing your posts.

Another sign that I follow, when building your network of friends, is to avoid people who have very few friends (meaning avoid acquiring them as friends if you don't already know them and/or they have a small social circle. If you personally know them, even if they have a lower number of friends, being personally associated with them can be more important than how many connections they have on social media).

Facebook allows up to 5,000 friends, but if someone has a lower number, like 250-350 friends this points to very little use of social media and the number of people who see your posts will be limited (through them). Or they haven't been on social media for very long. Think of the difference between having 2,000 friends who also have 2,000 friends and how much more exposure you'll get. Some people start a Facebook page thinking they want it but then never really get into it or find a way to utilize it for themselves (e.g. business, family, clubs, organizations, advertising, socializing, etc.).

Weed the garden refers to "refining" your group of friends once you have built it up to 5,000. *In the beginning, quantity is most important.* As you progress, the quality of the people is a higher priority. Refining represents fine-tuning to make connection with people you have more things in common with, which results in others taking a more emotional interest in your situation. Of course, this implies you show interest in them too!

How you go about this is by watching the posts, comments and responses your friends and acquaintances make to your and others' posts. For me, I look for people who have a positive mindset, positive attitude and are associated in some way to a healthy lifestyle. *Think about it.* Any one of your friends may become your actual living donor…you want healthier people, right? You want people who you can mutually lift each other up! Generally speaking, people who are overweight, don't exercise, smoke, do drugs, or are on a lot of medications will not qualify to help you regardless how enthusiastic they are anyway.

How you go about this is to gain information, from the first impression you get, from their Facebook picture. The first statement or quote under their picture tells you how they think and what's important to them…how do they live their life? What are their priorities?

If people seem to want to provoke, argue, prove a point, behave defensive, start disagreements or try to convince me my beliefs and values are wrong, I pass them by and if I befriend someone who does this after the fact, I delete them as a friend to make room for more positive people and people I have things in common with, even if it's just an attitude about life. When I started expanding my friend list, in January 2019, I had about 350 friends, most of whom I personally knew, many for my whole life. Sometimes there can be a stigma about friending a stranger, but overall, I haven't had any serious problems.

On Facebook, you can unfriend a person, you can block them, which means they can't find you on there anymore, nor see your posts or information anymore. If someone posts something offensive or explicit you can block them and report them to Facebook. I have had maybe 20 people, who once I friended them, they start sending explicit material within the messenger area of Facebook, where you can have conversations without the whole world seeing your conversations.

What I do with my posts looking for a kidney is to instruct others to message me privately, so our conversation isn't showing up publicly for everyone else to see. Keep the conversation confidential/private...*don't air your laundry!* Your posts are public, but once someone responds, conversations need to be private!

Part of how I screen people before requesting to be friends is by my **first impression** of their photo. **Secondly**, I look at what they write below their picture. This tells you about what they are most passionate about, interested in and their big-picture outlook on life. If you're into fishing, you'll notice other fishermen/women post a picture with a fish they caught. If they're into shooting, they'll likely have a photo of themselves with a gun. If they're a realtor, they'll likely have a very professional photo, etc.

After I read their opening statement below their picture, I scroll down a bit and click on, *"See Joe's about info."* This area is where you can see their interests, movies they like, clubs they're in, places they have been, what they do for work, their education, etc. This is another way to see how much you have in common with them. If they don't have anything in this info area, I'm not likely to friend them. Something may be "off".

After I look at their info, I scroll down a little further to "photos". On Facebook you can make numerous photo albums. By looking through a few of their photos you get a good feel for them and what they're about. If someone doesn't post any photos or only one, often they're up to something unscrupulous. It could possibly be they are being extra careful and private, but I've found rarely is that the case.

After looking at photos, I look at their last 20 or so posts. This is where you find out how positive they are and how well your values are similar to theirs. You get a good feel for them by looking at their posts.

I found that when I first started expanding my friend list, it took a lot more requests for connection than it did as my list grew. You have to realize that they are screening you too! Often, others are more resistant to accept friendship of people who have few friends. To some it looks suspicious because people who try to set up fake accounts often haven't been on long enough to make a lot of real friends or they make their friend list private so the public can't see their friend list or they have gotten so many denied friend requests that they don't have an extensive social group (this points to the fact they have probably been reported to Facebook for unscrupulous activity, were shut down, and now they're trying to get started again). Social, well balanced people generally like to connect with other social people!

Facebook also limits you to placing 1,000 friend requests at a time. This means if you put in 1,000 requests at once, you'll have to wait until some of them respond positively or deny you, to create more room for you to place more requests. As my own list of friends expanded, more and more people were faster to respond with a yes.

You might notice that as you're scrolling down through the newsfeed that everyone else's posts show up.

Usually Facebook posts suggestions of people who might be a good connection for you. When I'm connecting with people whom I've never seen before, I follow the steps I described above, but also send a message in Facebook messenger to them with a cartoonish likeness of me (also known as a sticker), usually me smiling and waving at them. Secondly, below the sticker I say something simple like, *"Love your posts!"*

The point of this is to build rapport with someone I don't know, as quickly as possible. That short statement is personal, but not so personal its invasive, so in this way its personal, but general. Knowing we don't know each other, I can't comment as if I know them. That would seem fake and superficial, which would be the opposite effect for making a fast-friend. By saying, *"Love your posts!"* it lets them know I looked at their page (taking an interest in **them).** If you don't send a personal message, they still might accept your friendship, but overall, I have found this to work better. I may even "like" two or three of their pictures before sending the request, again, to show I appreciate something **about them, which they are notified of.**

When I'm doing this, I'm not very attached to *which* people respond to my request, but rather making enough requests to meet my goal. No need to feel offended by those that don't accept your friendship…*it has no impact on the accomplishment of the overall, big-picture goal.* Some people only go on Facebook once-a-month…they're not going to respond quickly. Some people are on all day and have it set up with settings to get notifications instantly when you request friendship. I didn't keep track, but I estimate that in order to get 5,000 Facebook friends I made somewhere in the neighborhood of 15,000 requests, over the course of 15-months. And part of this number is based on deleting offensive people, argumentative people and people who think they can criticize and/or judge me for what I post on my own Facebook page. Truly, some people join Facebook just to try to start arguments with others...its a refection of their vales and how they choose to live their life. *-Avoid them like the plague!*

When you look at the list of comments, responses, requests by others to friend you and so on, you'll also see notifications of everyone who has a birthday on that day, if they have posted one in their profile. I make a point to wish everyone I'm a friend with a happy birthday. What I personally do, is wish every single person I'm associated with a happy birthday! In the messenger area of Facebook, you can send an electronic card, a gif, photos, messages, the list in endless. People love this! ***Again…taking an interest in them!*** These actions help your cause immensely and creates happiness for others. Every day I receive messages back saying I made their day, or it was the best birthday message they have ever received.

You can **post** it on their actual Facebook page, but everyone is doing that! Messenger, as long as they have it set up, and are using it, is more personal. If they don't have messenger set up, then I post to their page where everyone is posting. Often, a small icon changes color when they have viewed your message within messenger.

Notice the overall pattern of using Facebook is to *make quality connections that are win-win.* Show appreciation *for them*. Acknowledge *them.* Remember, this is not the platform for dumping your baggage or using others as a venting outlet. The more positive you truly are the better responses you'll consistently get! People like to help positive, abundant feeling people! The people who use social connections to dump/vent their emotional baggage, dump their anxiety and attempt to co-miserate have a much more difficult time acquiring volunteer donors, let alone friends. **Like-begets-like.** Abundance attracts abundance. Positivity attracts and inspires people.

People already assume you're suffering, they don't benefit from hearing about all the details. That's what prayer is for! People like to see others who are living a full life, making lemonade out of lemons and making the best of every situation. The more positive you are and communicate the easier it will be to build your list of living donors. Most people who need a kidney are fortunate to find one potential donor *in several years*. This can be discouraging, but you have power and control over it. People like to see you're doing as well as you can, making honest efforts, taking care of yourself and that they can potentially help you do even better…again, win-win. If you've ever been around chronic-complainers and noticed how tired you felt from having them go on and on about what's bad in life, bringing the conversation back to them and telling stories that help them feel better in the moment but doesn't contribute to you in any way. You know what I'm talking about. I've heard them referred to as time-gremlins or vampires…time gets taken up and essentially wasted but very little of anything productive comes of it. The show Saturday Night Live has hilarious characters based on this.

Even when we have a temporary challenge like being on dialysis and prepping for transplant, we have constant opportunities to improve the day of ***others.*** I estimate I've had near 200 doctors, nurses, psychologists, ultrasound techs, dieticians, nursing assistants, dialysis techs, social workers and on and on, during the last 21-months. With every single one of them, as long as I was actually conscious, I have worked to make them feel good in the moment…make their day somehow better…even if it's just asking them about what interests them! This in turn releases healing, soothing hormones in the body, which makes you feel better all on its own. The way I look at it, is that ***they are saving my life…I want to make their job as easy as possible***…I want them to have as pleasant of time as possible…they're giving up a part of their life to save mine! I tell them how much I appreciate them regardless of what's going on with me.

Ask them about their lives, just not as in screening their health or qualifying them…that's your transplant team's job!

Chapter Twelve

Create your own reasons to look forward to tomorrow.

One of the most powerful things you can do to make yourself feel better physically, mentally, emotionally and spiritually is to CREATE things (activities, experiences, travel, relationships, etc.), *to look forward to.* Research as shown that one's attitude can literally mean the difference between life and death. This is because of the multitude of mind~body connection(s) and the chemicals the brain and body simply produce, from looking forward to, imagining and projecting how bright your future can be affects health in tangible, physical ways. The opposite attitude literally produces the stress hormones cortisone and adrenaline, which literally break tissue down, interfere and sabotage healing and immunity.

Health care providers are acutely aware of each patient's attitude and this hints to the patients' likelihood of recovery and how well they respond to treatments. There's been a ton of research on this and its ongoing. You can find it on Google.

The emotional-state(s) affect which chemicals the body and brain are making. You can affect this process one way or the other…*its your choice.* The dichotomy is that most people think and live as if the emotions are something that "happens" [to them] without any control or influence over them (outside-in). In truth, the professionals who help people improve their life and effectiveness, on a daily basis, know that you can either let your emotions run you or you can take responsibility for them and create emotional states that empower you and make you feel better *more of the time*…affecting your overall outcomes (from the inside-out). People who leave their emotions to chance and "react" to the outside world tend to have more trouble, remain unhappier and struggle to find and sustain inner peace.

People who realize they have choice about how they "feel" emotionally and that they can create a consistent positivity state, tend to heal faster, have less infections and less hospitalization. Positive people are much easier for health care providers to help! *You want your team to look forward to seeing you, right!?*

Gratitude, and forgiveness tie into this as well. *Gratitude*…for anything, no matter how seemingly irrelevant, gets the mind on track for health, happiness and success. *Forgiveness* frees up mental, emotional, spiritual and physical energy (for what's important to you in present time), by permitting your spirit and mind to detach from the pain of the past, no matter how bad it was. A lot of people who have trouble getting what they want, in present time, have often been unwittingly/habitually delegating/permitting a portion of their energy to remain "feeding" the past…it's a lose-lose proposition…what you focus on grows and becomes a big part of your life as well as your identity, stealing intent, energy and emotions from what they want today. Getting something new, changing course, can take a lot of energy that we can't afford to split the emotional energy and focus between the past, present and future.

Practicing just these two principles, *gratitude and forgiveness,* have a huge impact on the body's ability to heal and recover efficiently.

Creating new (more useful in *this moment*), emotions is as easy as imagining what it is you want most, but instead of putting it off in the future, fully experiencing it as if its already done or accomplished (simply using your imagination for your own good to demonstrate to your mind where you want to end up). Some people say they will, *"...believe it when they see it,"* but how you get things done is to *believe it **until** you see it.*

Part of why this works is that the way the mind works is when you experience something as *done/complete*...the mind creates the emotions that create the behaviors to make the thing come to pass...*at an unconscious level,* outside your conscious awareness.

Practicing experiencing gratitude for the thing having happened assumes it has already occurred, which becomes a form of self-fulfilling prophecy, for lack of better term. This process takes energy and one who focuses on all the bad of the past is similar to a car with a leaking gas tank...*it's an unnecessary waste of useful resources*. It could also be compared to driving your car but trying to use the rear-view mirror to get where you want to go.

Chapter Thirteen

Change your emotional state from the inside out!

More often than not, the people who have a difficult time reaching their goals, regardless of the context, have been using their emotions efficiently, for their own good. Until taught, people generally believe that emotions "happen" "to them".

On the other hand, people who are used to achieving a positive attitude and reaching their goals have realized at some point that emotions are there for their use and it's our responsibility [to ourselves] to be aware of our emotional state and more importantly whether its not creating feelings we prefer.

The improvement of a more positive emotional outlook occurs inside the mind, *at will*. People who haven't yet realized they are in control of their emotional state(s) will often think that their emotional state is a side effect of what they just experienced, in the outside world. This is a big influencer for people who "can't lose weight" or improve their financial situations or living conditions. In other words, if they are grumpy, instead of going inside themselves and analyzing why they are having those feelings, they simply blame whoever is around them. Then, instead of resolving the feelings they do things to soothe themselves (self-medicate, in a sense), instead of resolving it. A lot of the time this might include lashing out on others, in weak attempt to feel better. Again…a temporary fix. They attribute their feelings to others (co-dependency). In the longer-term, this can contribute to a feeling of powerlessness and inability to achieve and have control over one's life. Overall, this metaphor is that, *"...life just happens to me,"* but it doesn't have to be that way.

In order to create a more positive, enjoyable and fulfilling life experience, a potential goal is to create an unconscious habit (through repetitive practice), of looking at the bright side, feeling better, having a brighter outlook, expecting good things to happen, expecting blessings and looking forward to a bright future…gratitude and forgiveness. This is essentially a practice of elevating your thoughts, to a realm "above the current situations".

A big part of developing this habit is practicing "remembering" times from the past when you had a great experience and felt really good, *even if it was just for a moment*. The reason being that because your mind has had that good experience, it can re-access it as a memory, repeat it, expand it and utilize it in current time as well as make it a habit outside awareness, so it doesn't require constant attention, which is what we all do anyway!

A person who has never had a great moment can just make one up, expand on it and build on it.

Once you remember a positive emotion, you then practice attaching the feeling to the thing you want, an experience you want or any other form of experience. By consistently practicing or "rehearsing" your success, regardless of the category, the mind starts to make connections in many ways (far beyond the scope of this brief book) which enable what you want to come about! If you want to do more research on this topic specifically, you can do a Google search of "future-pacing" which is the process I just described to you. There are several variations of this exercise/practice and you can experiment as well as fine tune it based on your goals. This technique is used worldwide by coaches to help people achieve their goals including professional and Olympic athletes, actors and actresses, musicians, politicians, elite military groups and so forth.

Any time you're working to accomplish something you've never experienced before, this process helps the mind comprehend what it is you want, (from an emotional standpoint, which is the most important influencer to the mind for achievement). Without the emotional aspect (of how good you feel getting or experiencing or achieving the thing), the mind doesn't understand the importance of it to you as a singular desire or goal.

Even the navy SEALS rely on this technique to help assure their success in some of the most demanding situations known. They refer to it as "rehearsing".

Rehearse your success!

Chapter Fourteen

Have something bigger than yourself.

Research has shown that when people reduce the focus on themselves and expand on helping others, everything seems to go better for everyone involved.

A person who is overly focused on how the world isn't fair, how much they're suffering, how they wish things were different will likely struggle to maintain physical, mental and emotional balance.

The people who look to improve the day of those around them will likely receive back more than they gave, which helps everything else!

I personally just try to help or improve one person's day each day. Sometimes I get lucky and am able to help three or four people or more in a day. The point is, what you put out or take comes back to you many-fold, so choose your daily approach carefully.

We can't control others (although a lot of people try), we can't control circumstances, but we can control what we perceive as the major themes in our life each day. We can also control our attitude which affects everything in our experience and our environment for better or worse.

Chapter Fifteen

Exercise and nutrition.

With exercise, I think we all know that people who exercise, within their current fitness level, feel better and do better in every context than people who do not exercise. I've been a personal trainer for 30-years, so I know it and have written several books on the topic, which are available on Amazon.

When I first got sick, I was so weak I could only lift a two-pound dumbbell, which I was using lying in bed, on my back, doing as many exercises as I could laying down. Again, in order to tell the mind and body what direction I intended to go in…*healing & vitality.*

I won't go into a long description nor exercise instruction here, I've already done that in my blog (listed in the *Appendix* on page 58), and previous books. But, I'll tell you that over the course of thirty-plus-years, a combination of resistance-training, also known as weight-training followed by 20-minutes riding a stationary exercise bike, is a very powerful combination. Not only staving off *de*-generative *dis*-ease, but preparing the body to simply do better overall, improving mental and emotional well-being and preparing the body for kidney transplant. The body simply bounces back much better when you have been exercising consistently, leading up to surgery. Exercise and proper nutrition (which is also included in my other books) balances body chemistry helping the lab tests be in a better range for good health.

Almost every lab test will improve from better exercise and nutrition, done within your current fitness level.

Many people don't feel as good on dialysis but simply doing what you can, exercise wise, is very important. It doesn't matter how little exercise you get because as the body adapts and gets stronger, you'll be able to consistently do a little bit more, up to about 4 ½ hours per week, resting a day between sessions. The ultimate goal, being 50-minutes of <u>moderate</u> weight-training followed by 20-minutes riding the stationary bike, three-times per week. If you can only do one minute of each that's fine, that's where you're starting from. If it takes you six-months or a year to build up to that, that's fine too!...you'll be making progress all along the way! AND, if you don't know what to do or how, get professional help.

If you ride the bike first, followed by the resistance-training, it has the opposite effect of benefits on physiology, metabolism, energy level and so forth…in other words, don't do it!

When I refer to weight-training or resistance-training, I'm talking about "moderate" amounts of weight, simply to get and keep the muscles working through a full range of motion. It's not a competition or lifting event to see how much you can lift, which would set you up for injury and likely setbacks, which you don't need.

MOST IMPORTANT is safety, which means using modern exercise equipment like at a commercial gym and getting professional training and instruction, to help assure you don't hurt yourself while trying to improve yourself!

I cannot overemphasize enough to GET PROPER EXERCISE INSTRUCTION BY A PROFESSIONAL PERSONAL TRAINER, who has been properly-trained to take your current health circumstances into account and takes your physical health into consideration.

In the 21-months leading up to transplant, I was very physically active, lifting weights, doing yard work, moving heavy things, and so forth. Once I knew an approximate surgery date, I increased my $_2$ exponentially, from doing 20-minutes three-times a week to doing up to 2-hours of cycling at a time (17 miles) three-times a week, even though I was anemic.

In addition, I made sure I had a good surplus of nutrition on board, in my body, so I would recover from dialysis and exercise as much as possible. In the 14-months leading up to transplant surgery I gained nearly 30-pounds of muscle preparing for the stress of surgery. I figured I would lose some weight after surgery and sure enough I lost 20-pounds in the three-weeks following surgery. The day after surgery I walked a mile and started back to lifting light weights in my recovery room. The 4th week after surgery I had put back on about 3-pounds of muscle and was using exercise tubing and light weight to improve my recovery. By the 4th month, I gained 25lbs.

As a side note, with my surgery, not only did they do the transplant, but I had double-inguinal hernia surgery 15-years prior. The surgeon said all that scar tissue in my lower abdomen was like a big patch of cement. They had to cut some away, grind it out of there and use the retractors, of course to keep it all pulled back during surgery. In addition, the surgeon said my abs were about 4-times thicker than most people, from all the abdominal exercises I had done and they had to cut through that too. The scar tissue from the hernia surgery had attached to my bladder, so they cut that away. The kidney they transplanted in me had gotten bruised when it was removed, so there was a hematoma on the surface of it.

Even with all these details, which led to a 5 ½ hour surgery, I exceeded all of the medical team's expectations and was released from the hospital the 3rd day following surgery. In other words, attitude + exercise + nutrition = faster, better, less complicated recovery.

Chapter Sixteen

Shield yourself from others' trauma-drama.

As you progress through your treatments, you'll come across no shortage of people who (for various known and unknown reasons) will want to dump their negative dialysis experiences on you. This can be detrimental and create unreasonable fears and expectations that affect outlook and attitudes.

I make it a rule to really not talk about my dialysis experiences, unless someone asks or it's a very close confidant like family or friends, not related to dialysis in any way.

Giving others the benefit of the doubt you could say they want to help others by telling their story, but if they aren't trained counselors or therapists they don't have any business assuming you'll have the same experience as them anyway. Everyone's experiences are unique even though there are some predictable commonalities.

People, as I described earlier, try to find times and opportunities to vent, complain, release emotions and get others to carry their emotions…often unwittingly at inappropriate times. These people need to do this with their professional social-workers, counselors and therapists and leave it at that. Spreading negativity, especially in the medical world helps no one. What a person expects to happen, based on what others have said can affect patient outcomes in big ways.

If it doesn't suggest positivity, build positive expectations in other patients and help them feel better, keep it to yourself. I've had other patients at the dialysis centers insist they want to "help me" and it turned out to be a dump-session for them to relieve themselves of past experiences. In no way was it to help me. If it leaves them feeling better they got it off their chest but causes anxiety, worry or fear in the person they or you are talking to, it was to help them, not you. That's what your social worker is for.

Its so easy to help others feel better, expect good things and feel more relaxed in their own processes…and remember,..*what you put out comes back in surprising ways*!

By the time, June 2020 rolled around,

my list of living, volunteer

donors had exceeded 100

and continued to grow from there.

I had transplant surgery September 23rd 2020 and

had 106 living donor volunteers by that time.

Page reserved for Afterword By Krista Standeford

Page reserved for Afterword By Krista Standeford

Page reserved for Afterword By Krista Standeford

Page reserved for Afterword By Krista Standeford

Page reserved for Afterword By Krista Standeford

Page reserved for Afterword By Krista Standeford

Page reserved for Afterword By Krista Standeford

Page reserved for Afterword By Krista Standeford

Page reserved for Afterword By Krista Standeford

Page reserved for Afterword By Krista Standeford

Page reserved for Afterword By Krista Standeford

Page reserved for Afterword By Krista Standeford

Appendix

Contact Information:

Sovereign Valentine

CFT, CET, Yft, SSC, SPN, Cft, GFI, SFI, EMR, CERT, CMCht, Reiki Master

Reasons or Results! Training Systems ©2020

e-mail: sovereignmv@gmail.com

Sov's blog:

https://sovereign-valentine.mykajabi.com/blog

Mona Smith

Certified Life Coach

Email. **Journey.Of.Purpose@outlook.com**

Donor Krista Standeford